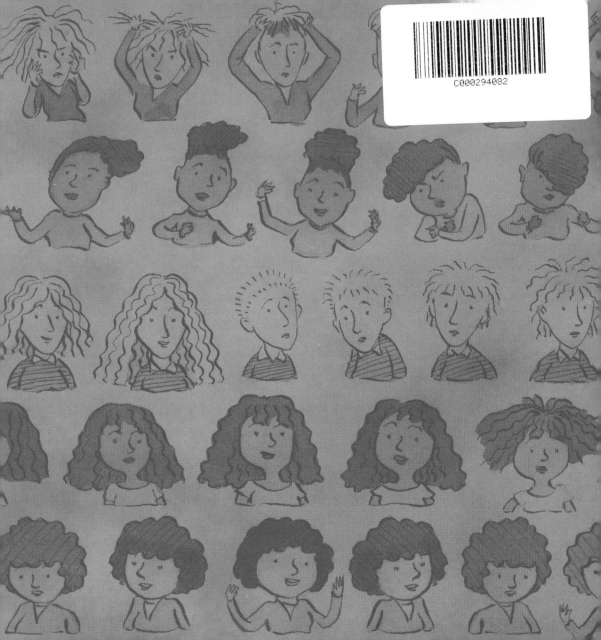

Philip Kingsley

Happy Hair Days

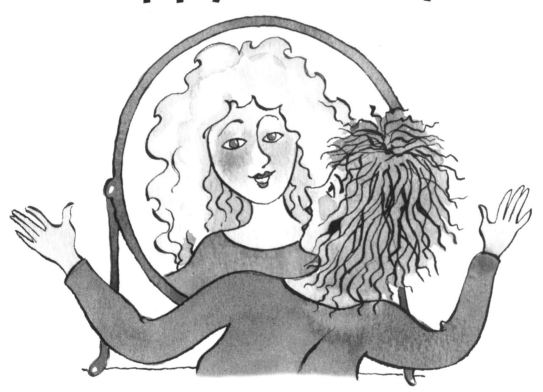

illustrations by Ian McNee

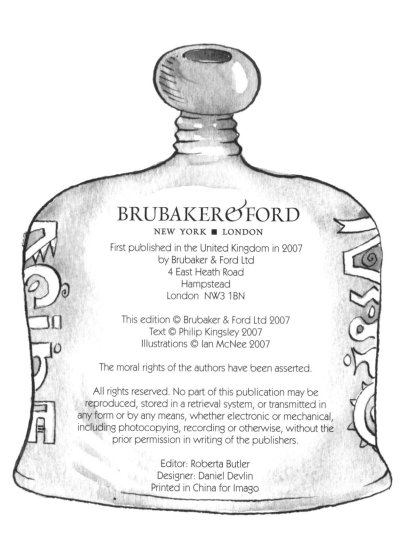

BRUBAKER&FORD

NEW YORK ■ LONDON

First published in the United Kingdom in 2007
by Brubaker & Ford Ltd
4 East Heath Road
Hampstead
London NW3 1BN

Editor: Roberta Butler
Designer: Daniel Devlin
Printed in China for Imago

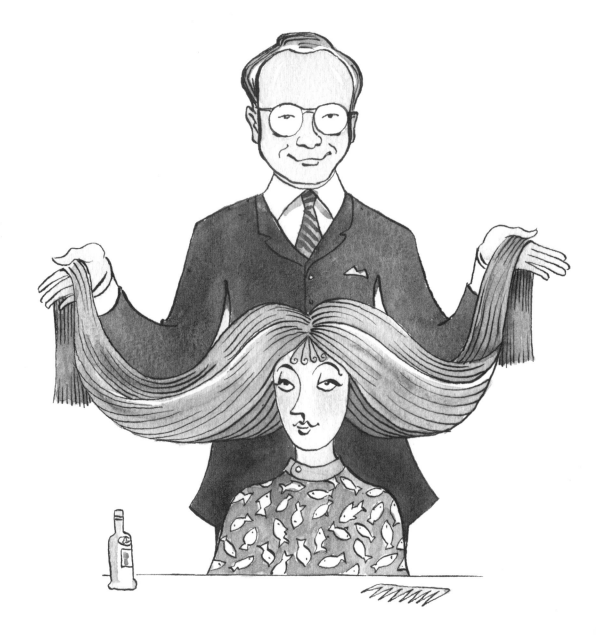

Similar questions and myths about hair care arise with an odd regularity. So much so that it seems many misconceptions have almost become folklore. These 50 Hair Tips address all of them. If you follow them (and why shouldn't you), they will lead to the Happiest Hair Days of your life.

What a wonderful way for me to celebrate my 50 years as a hair expert – one tip for each year!

Philip Kingsley

SHAMPOOING

Baby shampoos are specially formulated so as not to sting the eyes. But they are not better for your hair – or baby's. Quite the contrary. The best 'baby' shampoo is your own shampoo diluted: one part shampoo in four parts of purified water.

Shampoo your hair daily. You take your hair to the same places you take your face, and you know how dirty your face gets after a day!

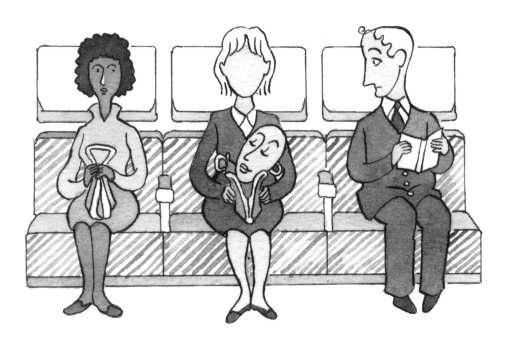

Using too much shampoo often causes dull hair. Soak hair with warm water, apply a little shampoo to the palms, spread over the hair, and massage gently. Add more water to increase lather. Rinse – and rinse again to ensure there is no residue.

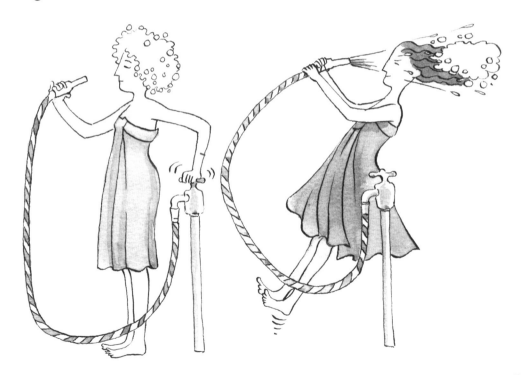

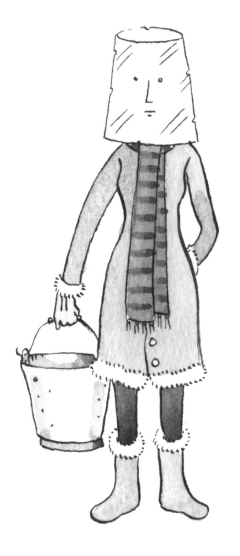

There is no scientific reason why a cold rinse should help your hair. In fact, it may even have the reverse effect.

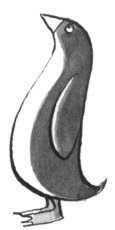

Scalp massage prior to shampooing can be beneficial. Place both hands on the scalp, fingers apart, and move the scalp over the skull in a circular movement.
One minute a day
is all you need.

Silicones in shampoos can be good, but too much can be detrimental. Look at the label: if the silicone (usually dimethicone) appears as one of the first three listed ingredients, choose another shampoo.

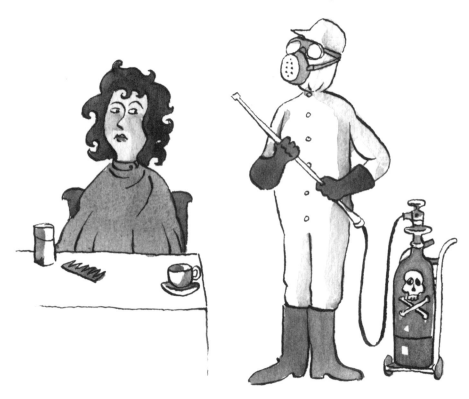

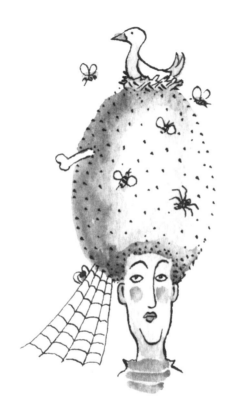

Rumour has it that if you don't wash your hair, it will cleanse itself. Utter nonsense! You should wash and condition your hair daily.

Don't expect too much from a shampoo. A shampoo
cannot work miracles. Think of your face: you cleanse
and you use many other cosmetics to make up.
Like your face, your hair needs other
'make-up' products. Use them
to create your own
Happy Hair Day!

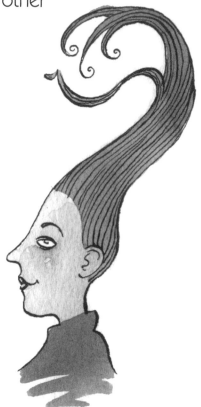

CONDITIONING

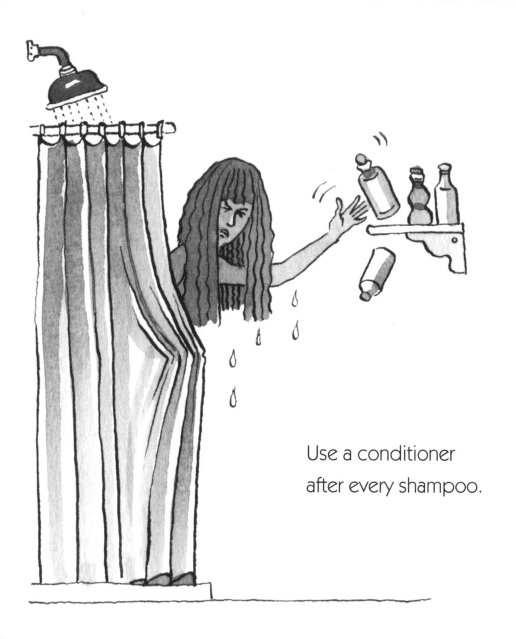

Use a conditioner
after every shampoo.

When detangling, start at the ends and gradually work your way up. Be gentle and NEVER start at the roots. Once all tangles are removed, then comb or brush from roots to ends.

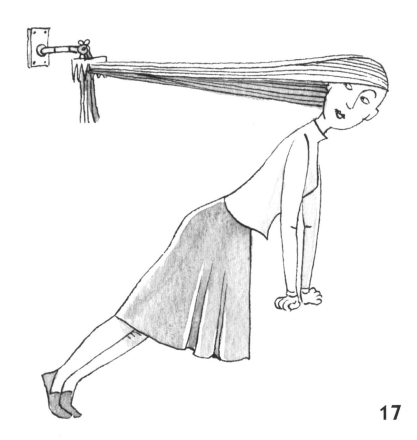

There is no such thing as 'overconditioning' your hair. Limp or dull hair results from using the wrong conditioner, or too much of it, or not rinsing properly – not from so-called 'overconditioning'.

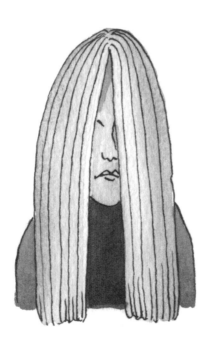

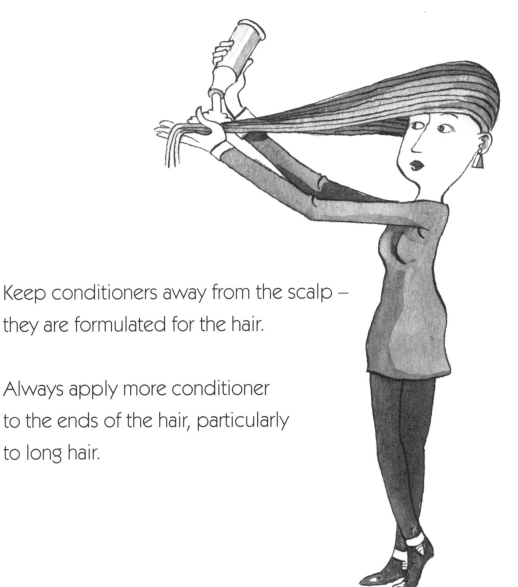

Keep conditioners away from the scalp –
they are formulated for the hair.

Always apply more conditioner
to the ends of the hair, particularly
to long hair.

Hair grows 6 inches a year. If it is 12 inches long, the ends will be 2 years old. So use more protective leave-in conditioner on the older and more 'weathered' ends.

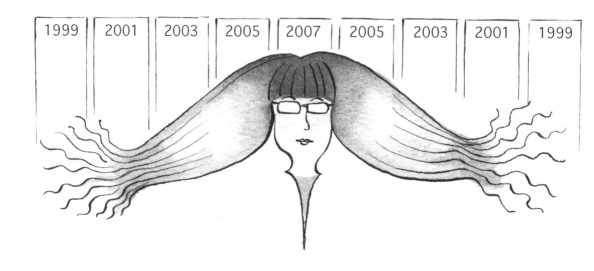

Whatever you read, whatever you do, you cannot heal a split end. The only way to cure split ends is to snip them off.

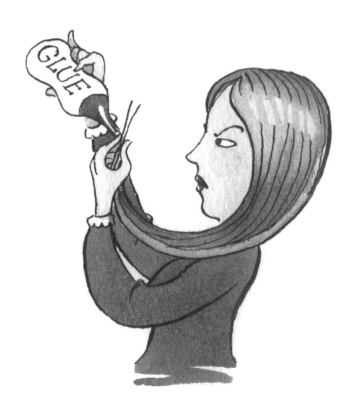

HAIR
PRODUCTS

There is no such thing as 'build-up' with hair products. Marketers selling 'clarifying' or 'build-up removing' shampoos would have you believe this myth.

Think of your face. You don't use a build-up remover to remove your make-up; you use a cleanser, or soap and water. Similarly, your regular shampoo will cleanse your hair of so-called build-up.

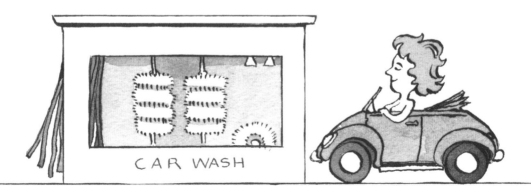

Deep-conditioning products are best used prior to shampooing. When done after shampooing, such products often leave the hair limp and unmanageable.

The old categories of 'Dry', 'Oily', or 'Normal' are no longer adequate for choosing hair products. They don't mean anything. For example, your normal is not my normal, or your friend's normal. The best hair products have a description on the label stating the type of hair they are for – read carefully and choose correctly.

Choose products according to your hair type: fine and limp, medium and wavy, coarse and frizzy, long or short, coloured or not.

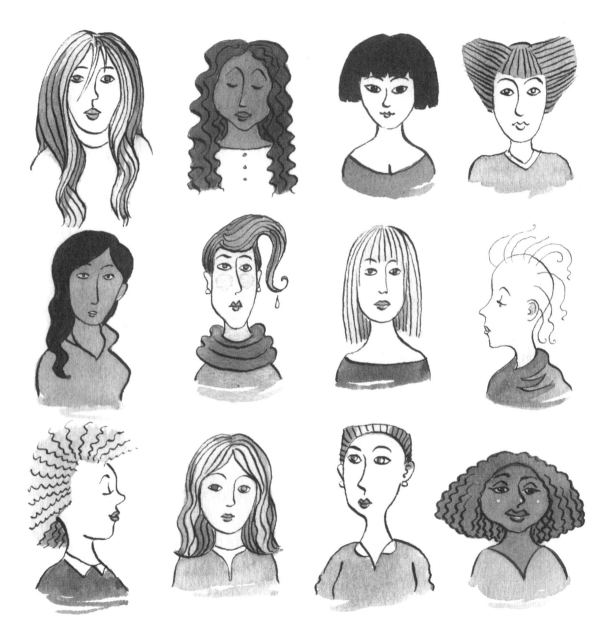

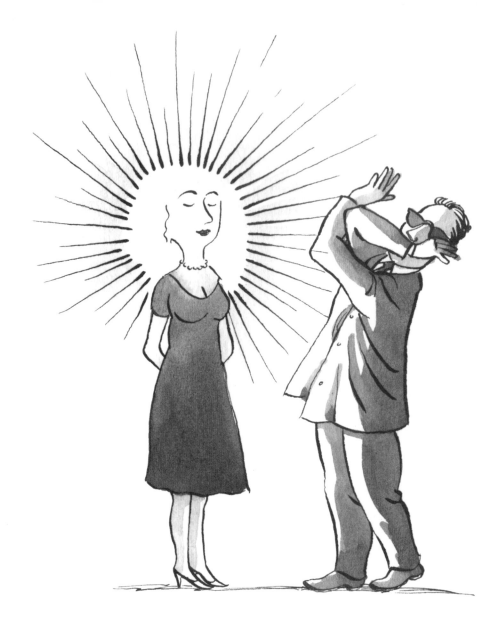

Shiny hair can be a sign of healthy hair. But shiny hair is only a reflection of light from the hair strands. Shiny hair has a smooth cuticle (outer layer). To attain this shine, use a conditioner. All conditioners help to smooth and flatten the hair's cuticle.

Healthy hair should stretch a third of its length before it breaks. If it doesn't, you need to use products that remoisturize and increase elasticity (stretchability). This is best done by hair treatment 'masks' that state they are formulated for this purpose.

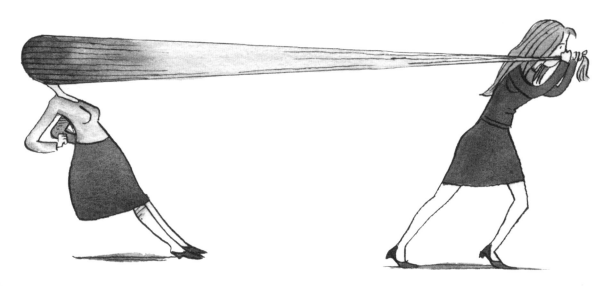

The terms 'natural' and 'herbal' are meaningless when applied to hair products. The more natural or herbal ingredients a product contains, the more 'unnatural' preservatives are needed to prevent spoilage.

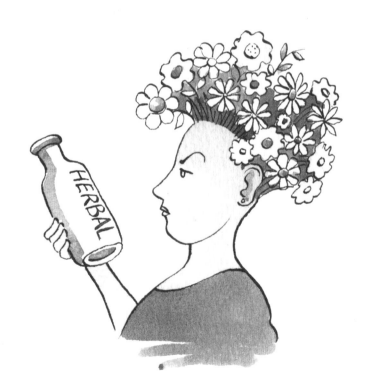

BRUSHING AND BLOW-DRYING

Correct blow-drying does not damage the hair. Just stop when your hair is dry; it is the blow-dryer on already dried hair that does the damage.

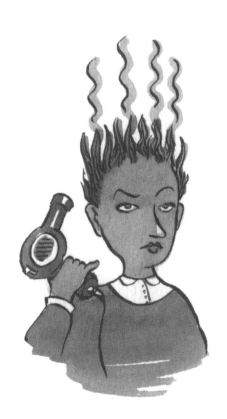

Don't brush your hair as an exercise – you'll pull it out and break it. Use a brush only to style, and when you do, be gentle.

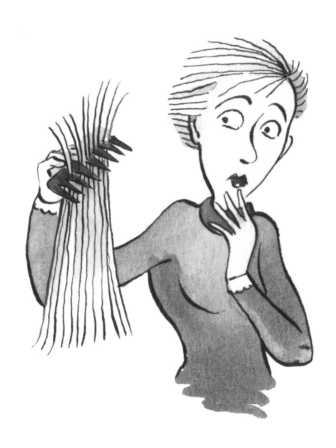

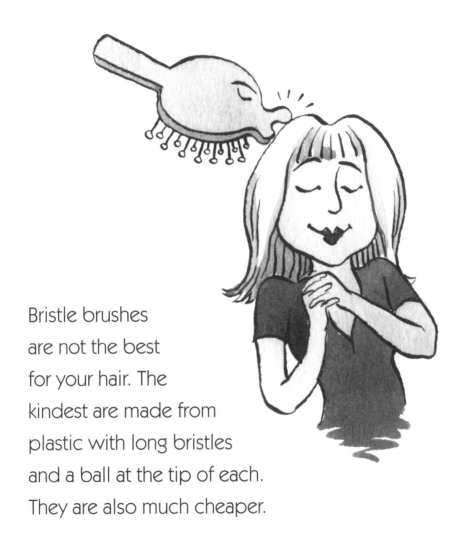

Bristle brushes
are not the best
for your hair. The
kindest are made from
plastic with long bristles
and a ball at the tip of each.
They are also much cheaper.

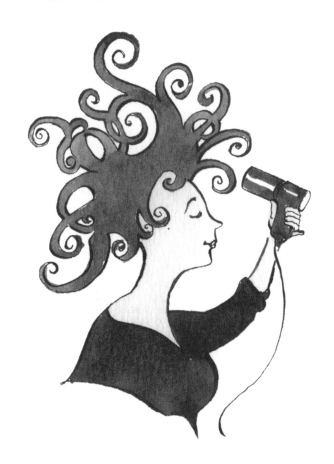

Use a protective styling aid before starting to blow-dry. Remember, though, that hot air will still penetrate the protection after your hair is dried.

To avoid split ends, apply a protective serum to the ends, and when blow-drying, hold the hairdryer at least 12 inches away.

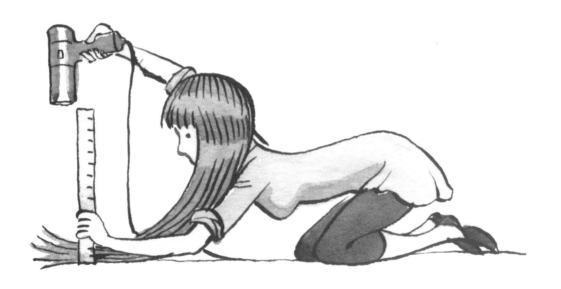

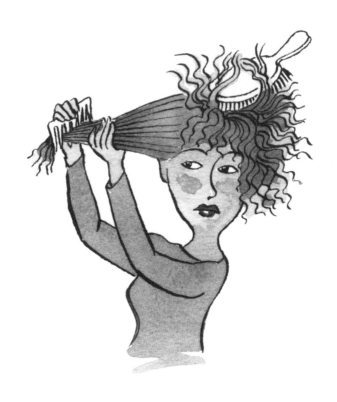

Detangle your hair with a wide-tooth comb –
not a brush.

DANDRUFF

Dandruff is **not** dry scalp. Dandruff is usually oily, so don't rub in oil to remove it – you'll only get oilier flakes.

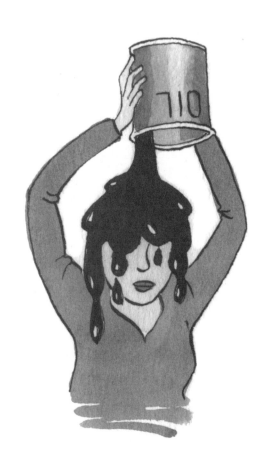

Do not confuse common dandruff with other forms of scalp flaking. If anti-dandruff shampoos do not help, visit your doctor; you may have psoriasis or eczema.

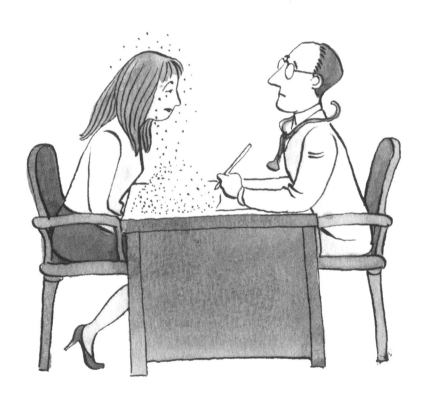

Stress often causes dandruff to worsen. A temporary measure to control dandruff is to shake together equal quantities of mouthwash and witch hazel and rub it into the scalp, before and after shampooing.

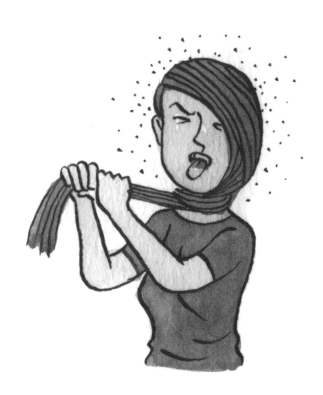

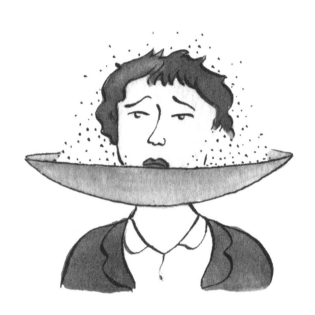

You cannot 'cure' dandruff forever. If you are prone to it (and over 70% of the population is), you can only **control** it. But modern shampoos, treatments, and tonics made for this purpose do so very effectively.

HAIR LOSS

There is no over-the-counter
hair-loss remedy. Don't waste
your money on trying them.

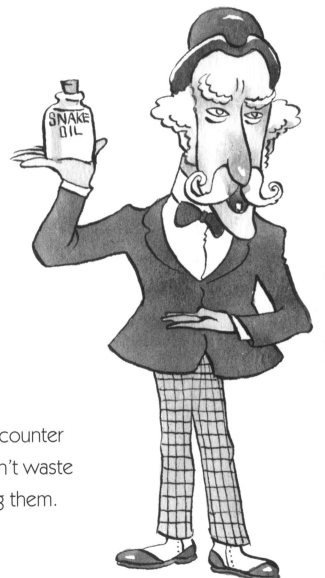

It is natural for hair to fall out – your whole head of hair is replaced every four years or so. You need only be concerned about hair fall if it increases over a long period, or if you notice your hair is thinner. There are seasons for extra hair fall: spring and autumn. This extra loss can last for four to six weeks, so don't worry if it does.

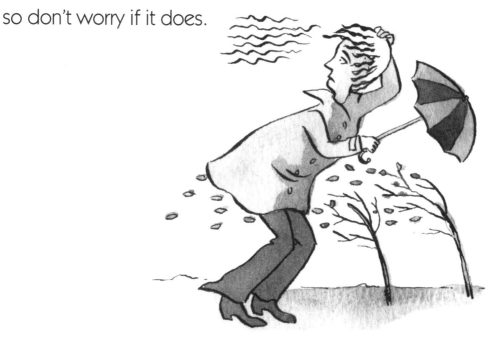

Most hair thinning occurs through diameter reduction. In other words, the hair gradually becomes finer in texture, making it seem thinner, but the number of hairs remains the same.

Hair loss usually results from a combination of circumstances. These could include nutritional deficiencies or excesses, low iron levels, and thyroid disturbances.

Ask your doctor to test for these, as well as for ferritin levels (iron stores), which aid hair cell renewal. It is not enough for ferritin to be 'normal'; it needs to be in the middle of the normal reference range for adequate hair follicle functions.

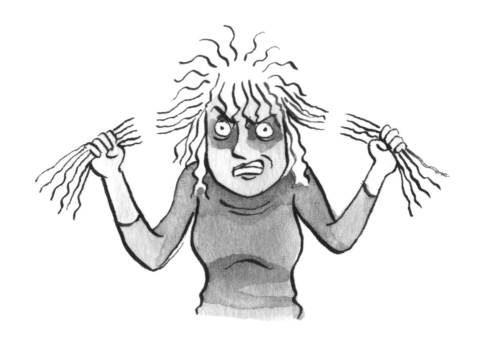

Stress is sometimes blamed for extra hair fall. This is
not a myth. Stress, through a convoluted route, can
produce more androgens, the male hormones that
can be responsible for hair thinning.

Lower your stress levels by meditation,
yoga, or an afternoon nap.

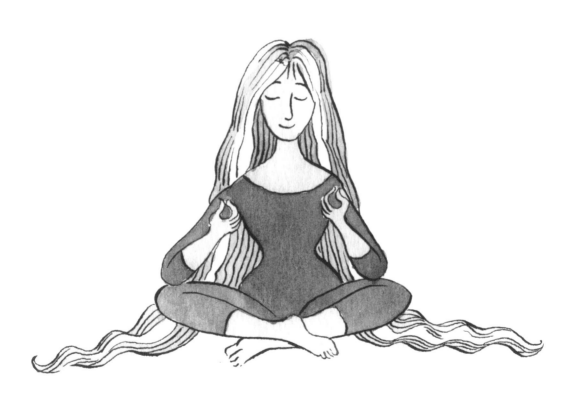

If your hair is thinning, look first to your diet. Hair consists of protein. A common cause of thinning hair is a lack of dietary protein. The most important meals for protein intake are breakfast and lunch. First class proteins for hair are meat, fish, fowl, eggs, and – to an extent – low-fat cottage cheese.

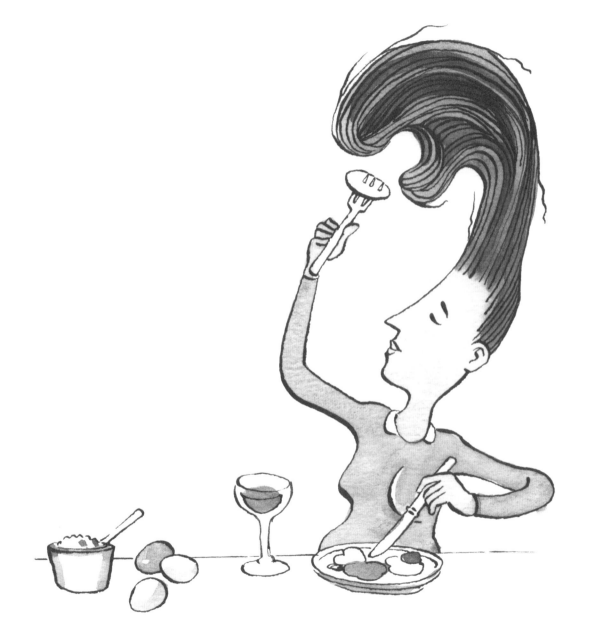

The energy to form hair cells diminishes four hours after eating a meal, so snack between meals to boost energy levels. The best energy-producing between-meal snacks for hair are complex carbohydrates, such as fruit.

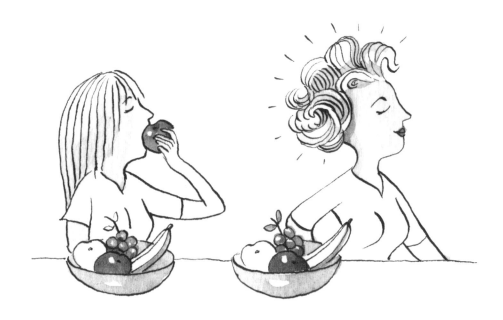

Cutting hair has absolutely
no effect on its rate of growth
or its strength.
Neither does shaving.

HAIR
COLOURING

There is no scientific evidence, nor physiological reason, why colouring hair makes it fall out or become thinner. If you want to colour, do so. Coloured hair, though, needs more care to prevent dryness.

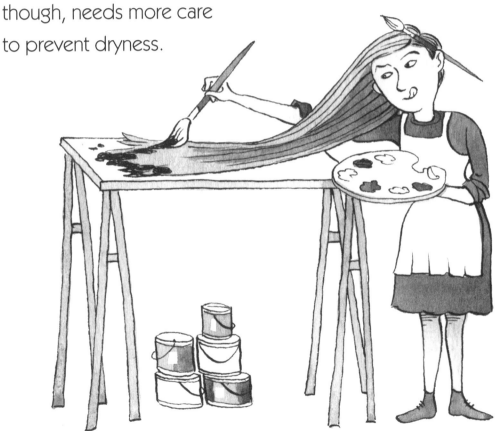

Many studies have concluded that there is no measurable risk of cancer from the use of personal hair dyes.

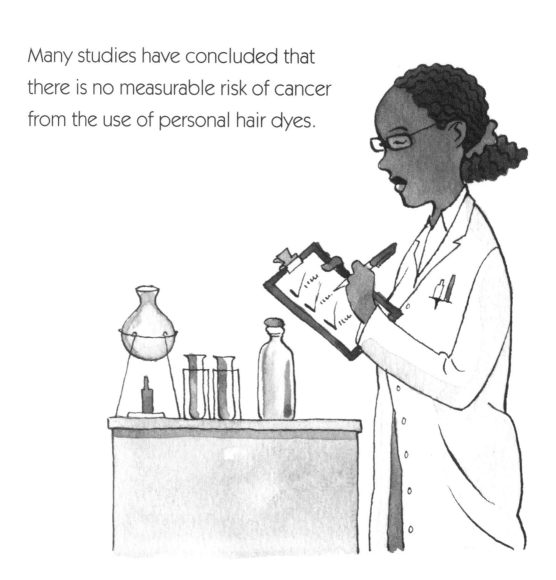

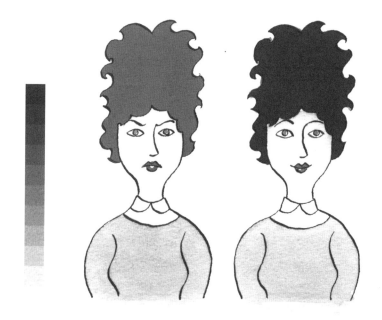

Many semi-permanent colours claim 'no peroxide' or 'no ammonia'. This is not quite as it sounds. There are other ingredients that have a similar effect with just slightly different names. And, anyway, semi-permanent colours do not give as good a cosmetic effect as do permanent colours. They fade more quickly and do not cover grey hair as well as permanent colours do.

If you think that permanent colours (or tints, or dyes as they are often called) are more harmful than semi-permanent dyes, think again. Remember that you will need to reapply the semi-permanent dye all over your hair every four to six weeks because it fades, whereas permanent colours only need to be applied to the roots. Due to overlap, when semi-permanent colour is reapplied, hair finishes up darker on the ends, which is the reverse of a 'natural' look.

Generally speaking, the lighter you colour your hair, the drier and more damaged it will become. Bleached and coloured blondes, for example, will have drier, more damaged hair than browns. However, if you like yourself blonde for Happy Hair Days, do it. Just condition and remoisturize more.

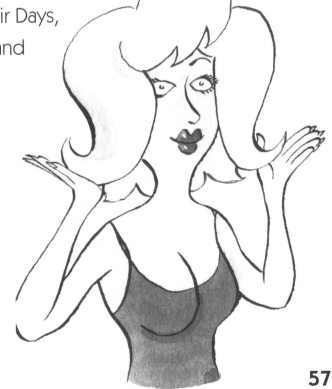

GREY HAIR

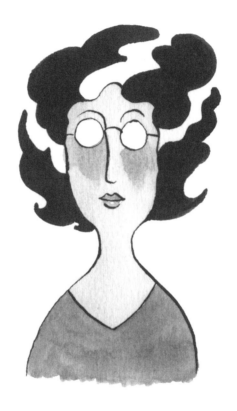

Grey hair is not coarser; it may be drier, which gives the impression of being coarser. Quite the contrary, it is usually finer. Hair does get finer as we get older.

When you pull out a grey hair,
two do not grow in its place.

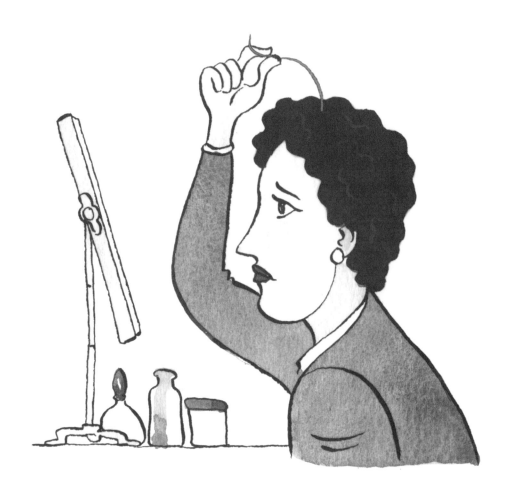

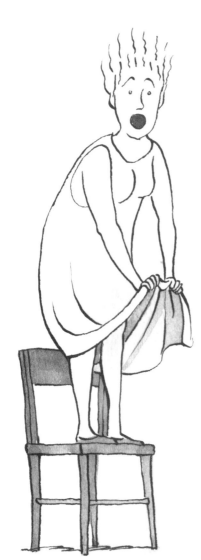

It is thought that Vitamin B levels influence greying of hair. Black-haired rats fed a diet deficient in B vitamins grew white hair. With replenished vitamin B, the hair regained its black colour. It has not been proven in humans, but anecdotal evidence suggests that large doses of the B vitamins may slow down greying, but not reverse it.

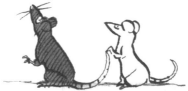

To avoid the yellow discoloration of grey hair, use styling aids with sunscreens, and avoid deep-coloured hair products, except those that are blue tinged.

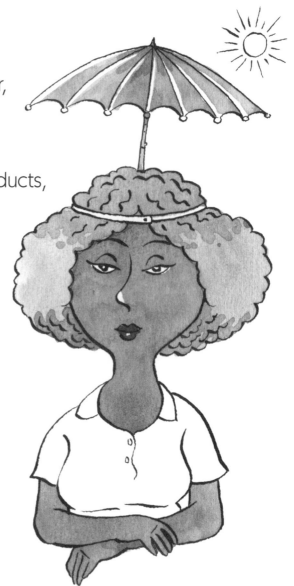

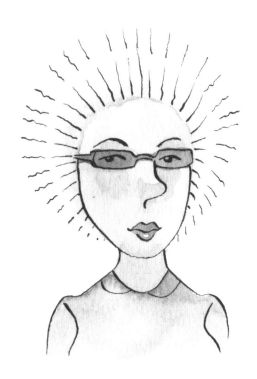

It may appear that grey hair is frizzier than before. This is because grey hair is drier and also finer. Dry hair tends to stick out; finer hair, not having the weight of thicker hair, doesn't lie in place as well either. Solve the problem by using a smoothing styling aid.

Well, there we are. I hope you have enjoyed
reading my 50 tips as much as I have
enjoyed compiling them. Above
all, I know that by following them
you will love your hair and have
Happy Hair Days like never before.

You know how your hair can
boost your morale (or the
reverse), so Happy Hair
Days mean happy days.
Enjoy them all –
along with your hair!

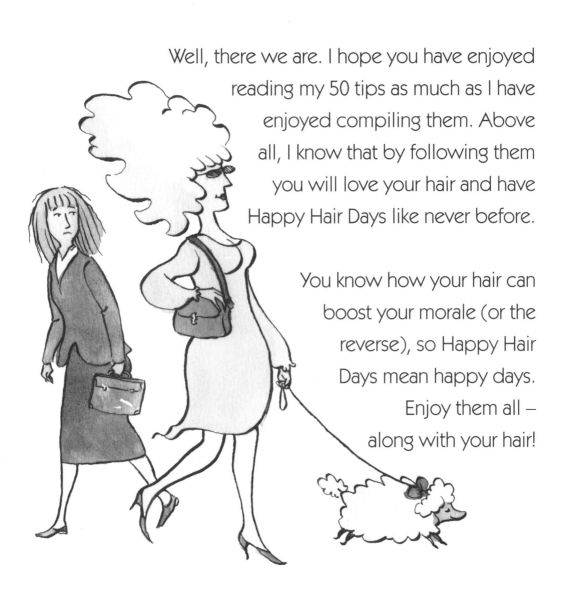

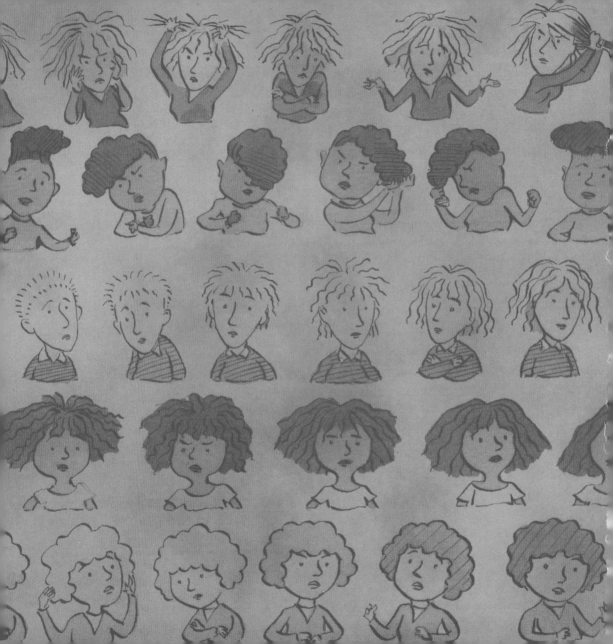